DEDICATION

To all the Little Warriors,

whose strength and resilience inspire us,

whose smiles light up our world,

and whose journeys with cerebral palsy

teach us the true meaning of bravery.

This book is dedicated to you,

as a guiding light on your path,

a source of knowledge and empowerment,

and a reminder that you are never alone.

May this book serve as a beacon of hope,

nurturing your dreams and aspirations,

and empowering you to overcome any obstacle.

You are the true warriors,

and your spirit shines brightly,

illuminating the world with your courage,

determination, and unwavering spirit.

With love and admiration,

Vanessa A. Ray.

TABLE OF CONTENTS

ACKNOWLEDGMENTS

Writing a book is a collaborative effort, and I would like to express my gratitude to all those who have contributed to the creation of "Little Warrior's Guide to Cerebral Palsy." Their support, expertise, and encouragement have been most valuable.

First and foremost, I would like to thank the little warriors themselves, the children and individuals with cerebral palsy, who have inspired me with their incredible strength, resilience, and unwavering spirit. Your journeys and stories have shaped this book and served as a constant reminder of the power of determination.

I would like to extend my deepest appreciation to the medical professionals, therapists, and researchers who have dedicated their careers to understanding and treating cerebral palsy. Your knowledge and expertise have provided the foundation for the information shared in this book.

To the families and caregivers who tirelessly support and advocate for their loved ones with cerebral palsy, thank you for your unwavering dedication and unconditional love. Your commitment to creating a nurturing and inclusive environment is truly commendable.

I am grateful to the organizations and support groups that work tirelessly to raise awareness, provide resources, and promote inclusivity for individuals with cerebral palsy. Your ongoing efforts have made a significant impact on the lives of countless individuals and families.

Lastly, I would like to express my heartfelt appreciation to my family and friends for their unwavering support and encouragement throughout this journey. Your belief in me and this project has been a constant source of motivation.

To all those who have played a part, big or small, in the creation of this book, thank you for joining me in empowering little warriors with cerebral palsy to live their lives to the fullest.

With gratitude,
Vanessa A. Ray.

1 UNDERSTANDING CEREBRAL PALSY: WHAT IT IS AND HOW IT AFFECTS YOU

INTRODUCTION

Cerebral palsy (CP) is a complex neurological condition that affects individuals from early childhood and throughout their lives. In this chapter, we will delve into a comprehensive understanding of cerebral palsy, its causes, types, and how it impacts various aspects of life. By gaining knowledge about CP, you will better be equipped to navigate its challenges and make informed decisions about your well-being.

Section1: Defining Cerebral Palsy:

1.1 What is Cerebral Palsy (CP)?

Cerebral palsy (CP) is a neurological condition that affects movement and posture. It is characterized by a group of disorders that causes varying degrees of physical disability. Unlike some other conditions, cerebral palsy is non-progressive, which means that the brain damage or abnormal development that causes it does not worsen over time.

CP is primarily caused by brain damage or abnormal brain development that occurs before, during, or shortly after birth. Brain damage or developmental abnormalities affects the parts of the brain responsible for controlling muscle movement and coordination. This damage or abnormal development can be a result of various factors, including parental and postnatal causes.

Prenatal causes of cerebral palsy include maternal infections, such as rubella or cytomegalovirus, exposure to toxins or certain medications during pregnancy, genetic disorders, and placental problems. These factors can disrupt the baby's brain's normal development, leading to cerebral palsy.

Perinatal causes of cerebral palsy refer to events or complications that occur during the birth process. Factors such as premature birth, oxygen deprivation(asphyxia), trauma during delivery, and complications like umbilical cord prolapse or placental abruption can lead to brain damage and subsequently result in cerebral palsy.

Postnatal causes of cerebral palsy can occur in the weeks or months following birth. These causes include severe head injury, infections such as meningitis or encephalitis, stroke, and certain medical conditions that affect brain development.

It's important to note that the specific causes of cerebral palsy may not always be identified in every individual case. Additionally, not all individuals with cerebral palsy have the same experiences or severity of symptoms. The effect of cerebral palsy can range from mild to severe and can impact various aspects of a person's life, including movement, coordination, speech and communication, sensory perception, and intellectual abilities.

While cerebral palsy is a lifelong condition, early intervention, therapies, and assistive devices can greatly improve the quality of life for individuals with CP. With proper support, individuals with cerebral palsy can achieve their potential, engage in daily activities, pursue education and careers, and actively participate in their communities.

1.2 Types of Cerebral Palsy?

Cerebral Palsy (CP) can be classified into different types based on the specific movement and muscle tone characteristics observed in individuals. The four main types of cerebral palsy are spastic, dyskinetic, ataxic, and mixed. Here's a description of each type and their primary symptoms and characteristics:

1. Spastic Cerebral Palsy:

   Spastic cerebral palsy is the most common type, accounting for approximately 70- 80% of all CP cases. It is characterized by increased muscle tone, resulting in stiff and tight muscles. The primary symptoms and characteristics of spastic CP include:

   - Spasticity: Muscles are stiff, and movements may be jerky or exaggerated.
   - Contractures: The tight muscles can lead to joint contractures, limiting the range of motion.
   - Scissors gait: Walking pattern characterized by legs crossing over each other.
   - Spastic diplegia or hemiplegia: in diplegia, both legs are affected more than the arms, while in hemiplegia, one side of the body is more affected than the other.
   - Difficulty with fine motor skills: Tasks such as writing or gasping objects may be challenging due to increased muscle tone in the hands and fingers.

2. Dyskinetic Cerebral Palsy:

   Dyskinetic cerebral palsy, also known as athetoid or dystonic CP, is characterized by abnormal, uncontrolled, and involuntary movements. The primary symptoms and characteristics of dyskinetic CP include:

- Involuntary movements: Movements may be slow, writhing, or twisting.
- Choreoathetosis: a combination of involuntary, purposeless movements (chorea) and abnormal, slow, writhing movement (athetosis).
- Dystonia: Sustained or repetitive muscle contractions cause twisting or contorted postures.
- Difficulty with coordination: Impaired control over voluntary movements, affecting tasks like reaching or grasping objects.
- Speech difficulties: Involuntary movements of the mouth, tongue or throat can impact speech clarity.

3. Ataxic Cerebral Palsy:

   Ataxic cerebral palsy is the least common type, accounting for approximately 5-10% of CP cases. It is characterized by problems with coordination and balance. The primary symptoms and characteristics of ataxic CP include:

   - Unsteady gait: Difficulty maintaining balance and coordination while walking.
   - Tremors: shaking or trembling movements, particularly during intentional actions.
   - Lack of precision and control: difficulty with fine motor skills, such as writing or buttoning clothing.
   - Hypotonia: Low muscle tone, resulting in poor muscle strength and control.
   - Instability: Difficulty with tasks that require precise movements or balancing, such as reaching for objects.

4. Mixed Cerebral Palsy:

   Mixed cerebral palsy refers to a combination of two or more types of CP. For example, an individual may exhibit characteristics of both spastic and dyskinetic CP. The primary symptoms and characteristics of mixed CP depend on the types present and can vary from person to person.

   It is important to note that individuals may have different degrees of severity and unique combinations of symptoms within each type of cerebral palsy. Proper diagnosis and assessment by healthcare professionals are essential for understanding the specific type and characteristics of cerebral palsy in an individual, which can guide treatment and support strategies tailored to their needs.

Section 2: Causes and Risk Factors:

2.1 Prenatal causes:

Prenatal factors play a significant role in contributing to the development of cerebral palsy (CP). These factors can affect the development of the baby's brain during pregnancy, leading to the manifestation of CP. Here's a discussion of some common prenatal factors that can contribute to the development of CP:

1. Maternal Infections:

   Certain infections contracted by the mother during pregnancy can increase the risk of cerebral palsy in the child. Examples of such infections include:

   - Rubella (German measles): Rubella infection during early pregnancy can cause severe developmental abnormalities in the baby's brain, leading to CP.
   - Cytomegalovirus(CMV): CMV is a common viral infection that can cause brain damage if transmitted from the mother to the fetus during pregnancy.
   - Toxoplasmosis: Infection with the Toxoplasma gondii parasite can increase the risk of CP if contracted during pregnancy.

2. Genetic Abnormalities:

   Certain genetic abnormalities or mutations can result in abnormal brain development, increasing the risk of cerebral palsy. These genetic factors can be inherited from parents or occur spontaneously during fetal development. Some genetic conditions associated with an increased risk of CP include:

   - Chromosomal abnormalities (e.g., Down syndrome, Turner syndrome)
   - Genetic disorders affecting brain development (e.g., tuberous sclerosis, fragile X syndrome)

3. Placental problems:

   The placenta plays a crucial role in supplying oxygen and nutrients to the developing fetus. Any disruptions or abnormalities in the placenta's functioning can potentially affect the baby's brain development, increasing the risk of CP. Placental problems that can contribute to CP include:

   - Placental abruption: premature separation of the placenta from the uterine wall, leading to oxygen deprivation and potential brain damage.

- Placental insufficiency: Reduced blood flow and inadequate oxygen and nutrient supply to the fetus, affecting brain development.

4. Maternal Health Conditions:

   Certain maternal health conditions can increase the risk of cerebral palsy in the baby. These conditions may affect the developing fetus directly or indirectly through their impact on maternal health. Examples include:

   - Maternal seizures or epilepsy: seizures during pregnancy can affect the oxygen supply to the fetus, potentially leading to brain damage and CP.
   - Maternal thyroid disorders: untreated or poorly controlled thyroid disorders in the mother can impact fetal brain development.
   - Maternal diabetes: poorly controlled diabetes during pregnancy can increase the risk of CP in the baby.

     It is important to note that while these prenatal factors can contribute to the development of cerebral palsy, not all cases of CP have identifiable prenatal causes. Additionally, the presence of these factors does not necessarily mean that CP will occur. The interplay between genetic predispositions, prenatal factors, and other unknown factors contributes to the complex nature of cerebral palsy's etiology.

2.2 Perinatal causes:

Perinatal factors refer to events or complications that occur during the birth process or shortly after birth. These factors can increase the risk of cerebral palsy (CP) by causing brain damage or abnormalities during a critical period of development. Here's an explanation of some perinatal factors associated with CP:

1. Birth Complications: Complications during labor and delivery can

   potentially lead to brain damage and increase the risk of CP. These complications may include:

   - Prolonged labor: Extended labor can cause oxygen deprivation or other stresses on the baby's brain.
   - Difficult or abnormal presentation: If the baby is not positioned optimally during delivery, such as breech presentation, it can increase the risk of birth

complications.

- Umbilical cord complications: Issues such as umbilical cord prolapse, compression, or a tangled cord can disrupt blood and oxygen flow to the baby's brain.
- Trauma during delivery: Injuries to the baby's head or brain during a forceps or vacuum extraction delivery can lead to CP.

2. Premature Birth:

Premature birth, defined as birth before 37 weeks of gestation, is a significant risk factor for cerebral palsy. Babies born prematurely are at higher risk of CP due to the following reasons:

- Immature brain development: The brain undergoes rapid growth and development during the final weeks of pregnancy. Premature birth interrupts this critical phase, increasing the vulnerability of the brain to injury.
- Increased likelihood of other complications: Premature babies may experience oxygen deprivation, intraventricular hemorrhage (bleeding in the brain), or infection, which can lead to CP.

3. Oxygen Deprivation (Asphyxia):

Lack of oxygen during or immediately following birth, known as birth asphyxia or hypoxic-ischemic encephalopathy (HIE), can cause brain damage and contribute to the development of CP. Oxygen deprivation can occur due to several reasons:

- Placental abruption: Premature separation of the placenta from the uterine wall can disrupt the oxygen supply to the baby.
- Uterine rupture: A tear in the uterus during labor can cause severe oxygen deprivation.
- Umbilical cord problems: Cord compression, knotting, or prolapse can obstruct oxygen flow to the baby.
- Respiratory issues: Difficulties in establishing breathing after birth, such as meconium aspiration or respiratory distress syndrome, can lead to oxygen deprivation.

It's important to note that not all birth complications, premature births, or cases of oxygen deprivation lead to cerebral palsy. The severity and duration of the event, as well as the individual baby's resilience, are determining factors. Prompt medical intervention and appropriate neonatal care can help mitigate the risks associated with perinatal factors and minimize the potential for brain injury and subsequent development of CP.

2.3 Postnatal causes:

Postnatal causes of cerebral palsy (CP) refer to events or conditions that occur in the weeks or months following birth and can contribute to the development of CP. These causes can result in brain damage or abnormalities, leading to the manifestation of CP. Here's an identification of some common postnatal causes of CP:

1. Traumatic Brain Injury (TBI):

   Traumatic brain injury refers to an injury to the brain caused by an external force. Postnatal traumatic brain injury can occur due to accidents, falls, physical abuse, or other incidents that result in head trauma. Severe head injuries can lead to brain damage and subsequent CP.

2. Infections:

   Certain infections that affect the brain can contribute to the development of CP. These infections include:

   - Meningitis: Inflammation of the membranes surrounding the brain and spinal cord can cause brain damage if not promptly treated.
   - Encephalitis: Inflammation of the brain tissue itself, often caused by viral infections, can result in brain injury and increase the risk of CP.

3. Medical Conditions Affecting Brain Development:

   Certain medical conditions can impact brain development, potentially leading to CP. These conditions include:

   - Genetic disorders: Certain genetic conditions affect brain development and can increase the risk of CP. Examples include tuberous sclerosis, neurofibromatosis, and metabolic disorders.
   - Metabolic disorders: Disorders that affect the body's ability to process nutrients or

remove waste products can lead to brain damage and CP.

- Brain tumors: Tumors in the brain can cause pressure, damage, or disrupt the normal development of the brain, resulting in CP.

4. Stroke:

Stroke refers to the interruption of blood supply to the brain, leading to brain damage. Postnatal strokes, although less common than strokes in adults, can occur in newborns or infants and contribute to CP. Strokes may be caused by blood clots, bleeding, or vascular malformations.

5. Hypoxic-Ischemic Encephalopathy (HIE):

HIE can also occur Postnatally, usually due to severe oxygen deprivation. Events such as near-drowning, suffocation, or prolonged respiratory distress can lead to HIE and subsequent brain damage, potentially resulting in CP.

It's important to note that not all postnatal causes of CP are preventable, and sometimes the specific cause may not be identified. Prompt medical attention, early diagnosis, and appropriate treatment of infections, medical conditions, or traumatic events are crucial in minimizing the risk of brain injury and subsequent development of CP.

2.4 Risk Factors:

Certain risk factors have been identified that may increase the likelihood of developing cerebral palsy (CP) in individuals. These risk factors can help healthcare professionals identify infants who may be at higher risk and provide appropriate care and interventions. Here are some key risk factors associated with CP:

1. Low Birth Weight:

Low birth weight, typically defined as weighing less than 2,500 grams (5.5 pounds) at birth, is a significant risk factor for CP. Premature infants are more likely to have low birth weight, and their immature organs, including the brain, may be more vulnerable to damage or abnormalities that can lead to CP.

2. Multiple Births:

The birth of twins, triplets, or higher-order multiples (such as quadruplets) is associated with a higher risk of CP compared to single births. Multiple pregnancies, especially those involving premature or low birth weight infants, can increase the chances of CP due to the higher likelihood of complications during pregnancy, labor, or delivery.

3. Maternal Health Issues:

Certain maternal health issues can increase the risk of CP in the baby. These health issues may include:

- Infections during pregnancy: Maternal infections, such as rubella, cytomegalovirus (CMV), or certain sexually transmitted infections, can pose a risk to the developing baby's brain, potentially leading to CP.
- Maternal medical conditions: Conditions like high blood pressure (hypertension), thyroid disorders, diabetes, or autoimmune disorders can increase the risk of CP if not properly managed during pregnancy.
- Substance abuse: Prenatal exposure to drugs or alcohol can cause significant harm to the developing baby, including brain damage that may result in CP.

4. Birth Complications:

Complications during labor and delivery can increase the risk of CP. Some examples of birth complications include prolonged labor, fetal distress, breech presentation, umbilical cord complications, and trauma during delivery. These complications can result in oxygen deprivation or trauma to the baby's brain, leading to CP:

5. Previous Sibling with CP:

Having a sibling with CP increases the likelihood of another child in the family being diagnosed with CP. Although the specific mechanisms behind this association are not fully understood, it suggests that genetic or environmental factors within the family may play a role in the development of CP.

It's important to note that the presence of these risk factors does not guarantee that CP will occur. Many individuals with CP do not have any identifiable risk factors, and conversely, not all individuals with risk factors will develop CP. Each case is unique, and multiple factors can contribute to the development of CP. Early identification of risk factors, along with appropriate prenatal care, monitoring, and intervention, can help mitigate the risks and improve outcomes for at-risk infants.

Section 3: Impact on Motor Function:

3.1 Motor Impairments:

Cerebral palsy (CP) is characterized by a wide range of motor impairments that can significantly impact an individual's mobility, fine motor skills, and activities of daily living. The three primary types of motor impairments associated with CP are muscle stiffness (spasticity), involuntary movements (dyskinesia), and lack of coordination (ataxia). Let's examine each of these impairments and their effects in more detail.

1. Muscle Stiffness (Spasticity):

   Spasticity is the most common motor impairment seen in individuals with CP. It is characterized by increased muscle tone, causing stiffness and resistance to movement. Spasticity affects both the agonist and antagonist muscles, leading to muscle imbalance and abnormal posture. Key effects of spasticity include:

   - Limited range of motion: Increased muscle tone restricts joint movement, making it difficult for individuals to perform activities that require a full range of motion.
   - Contractures: Prolonged spasticity can lead to the shortening of muscles and tendons, resulting in joint contractures. This further restricts movement and can cause joint deformities.
   - Impaired motor control: The increased muscle tone makes initiating and controlling voluntary movements challenging, leading to difficulties with coordinated actions.

2. Involuntary Movements (Dyskinesia): Dyskinesia refers to involuntary, uncontrolled movements that can be slow, writhing, or jerky in nature. These movements can be unpredictable and vary in severity. Key effects of dyskinesia include:

   - Lack of precision: The involuntary movements interfere with fine motor control, making tasks requiring precision and coordination challenging. Activities such as writing, buttoning clothes, or feeding oneself can be difficult.
   - Difficulty with posture and balance: Dyskinesia can affect trunk control

and balance, leading to difficulties in maintaining an upright posture and stability during movement.

3. Lack of Coordination (Ataxia): Ataxia is characterized by a lack of coordination and control of voluntary movements. It affects balance, spatial awareness, and the ability to perform smooth, coordinated motions. Key effects of ataxia include:

   - Unsteady gait: Individuals with ataxia often have an unsteady, wide-based gait, making walking and navigating uneven surfaces difficult.
   - Difficulty with fine motor skills: Ataxia can affect fine motor skills, such as precise hand movements required for activities like writing, typing, or using utensils.
   - Challenges with coordination: Coordinating simultaneous actions of multiple muscle groups, such as reaching and grasping, can be problematic due to impaired motor planning and execution.

3.2 Functional Limitations:

Cerebral palsy (CP) is a neurological disorder that affects movement, posture, and muscle coordination. The functional limitations experienced by individuals with CP can vary widely, depending on the severity and type of the condition. While CP primarily affects motor skills, it can also be associated with cognitive impairments, communication difficulties, and sensory issues.

- Walking: One of the major challenges faced by individuals with CP is walking. The ability to walk independently may be affected due to muscle stiffness (spasticity), muscle weakness, balance problems, or coordination issues. Some individuals may require assistive devices such as canes, walkers, or crutches to aid in walking. In more severe cases, a wheelchair may be necessary for mobility. Rehabilitation therapies, such as physical therapy and gait training, play a crucial role in maximizing walking ability by improving muscle strength, flexibility, balance, and coordination.
- Sitting and Standing:

  Individuals with CP may have difficulties with sitting and maintaining an upright posture due to muscle tone abnormalities. Muscle stiffness or weakness can affect their ability to control their body position and maintain balance while sitting. Additionally, standing may be challenging due to impaired muscle control and balance. Adaptive seating systems and postural supports can assist individuals in maintaining a stable and comfortable sitting position. Physical and occupational therapies can help improve trunk control, postural stability, and overall sitting and standing abilities.

- Manipulating Objects:

CP can affect fine motor skills, making it challenging to manipulate objects with precision and coordination. Difficulties may arise in tasks such as grasping, reaching, and manipulating small items. Occupational therapy can help individuals with CP develop strategies to improve hand-eye coordination, dexterity, and fine motor skills. Adaptive devices such as specialized utensils, writing aids, and computer accessibility tools can further enhance independence and assist in overcoming limitations while manipulating objects.

- Rehabilitation Therapies and Assistive Devices:

Rehabilitation therapies, including physical therapy, occupational therapy, and speech therapy, are essential for individuals with CP to optimize their independence and mobility. Physical therapy focuses on improving gross motor skills, strength, balance, and mobility, while occupational therapy addresses fine motor skills, self-care tasks, and activities of daily living. Speech therapy helps individuals with CP overcome communication challenges.

Assistive devices and technologies play a vital role in supporting individuals with CP. These can include mobility aids (wheelchairs, walkers), orthotic devices (braces, splints), communication devices (augmentative and alternative communication tools), adaptive seating systems, and specialized assistive technology for writing, typing, and computer access. These devices and technologies can enhance functional abilities, promote independence, and improve overall quality of life.

It is important to emphasize that each individual with CP is unique, and their specific needs and functional limitations can vary. An individualized approach to rehabilitation, including a comprehensive assessment and ongoing support, is crucial to maximize independence, mobility, and overall well-being for individuals with CP.

Section 4: Associated Challenges:

4.1 Communication and Speech Difficulties.

Individuals with cerebral palsy (CP) may face various speech and communication challenges due to motor impairments that affect the muscles used for speech production. These challenges can range from mild to severe, depending on the type and severity of CP. Some common speech and communication difficulties experienced by individuals with CP include:

1. Articulation difficulties: Muscle stiffness (spasticity) or weakness can affect the coordination and control of the muscles involved in speech production, resulting in unclear or distorted speech sounds.
2. Dysarthria: CP can cause dysarthria, a motor speech disorder characterized by slurred or slow speech, imprecise articulation, and difficulties with voice control and breath support.
3. Apraxia of speech: Some individuals with CP may also experience apraxia of speech, a neurological condition that affects the ability to plan and execute the precise movements required for speech production.
4. Voice disorders: CP can lead to voice disorders, such as hoarseness, breathiness, or a monotone voice, due to muscle tone abnormalities and difficulty controlling vocal fold tension.

To overcome these challenges and facilitate effective communication, alternative and augmentative communication (AAC) methods and therapies can be employed. These methods and therapies include:

1. Augmentative and Alternative Communication Devices: AAC devices range from low-tech options like communication boards or picture-based communication systems to high-tech solutions such as speech-generating devices

and tablet-based applications. These devices allow individuals to express themselves by selecting symbols, pictures, or words to form messages.

2. **Sign Language:** Some individuals with CP may benefit from learning sign languages, such as American Sign Language (ASL) or a modified version of sign language, to enhance their ability to communicate. Sign language can be used independently or in conjunction with other AAC methods.
3. **Visual Supports:** Visual supports such as communication charts, picture schedules, and visual cues, can assist individuals with CP in understanding and conveying messages. Visual supports can aid comprehension, promote independence, and facilitate communication in various settings.
4. **Speech Therapy:** Speech therapy plays a crucial role in helping individuals with CP improve their speech and communication skills. Speech-language pathologists work with individuals to address specific challenges, improve articulation, enhance voice control, and develop strategies to overcome difficulties with speech production.
5. **Oral Motor Exercises:** Oral motor exercises are designed to strengthen the muscles used for speech production. These exercises can help improve speech clarity and coordination by targeting specific muscle groups involved in articulation and breath control.
6. **Communication Strategies:** Speech-language pathologists can work with individuals with CP to develop effective communication strategies, such as using shorter sentences, employing gestures or facial expressions, and incorporating pauses to allow for processing time.

It is important to note that AAC methods and therapies should be tailored to the individual's unique needs and abilities. A multidisciplinary approach involving speech-language pathologists, occupational therapists, and assistive technology specialists can ensure comprehensive assessment, intervention, and ongoing support to maximize communication abilities for individuals with CP.

4.2 Sensory and Perception Issues.

Cerebral palsy (CP) is a neurological condition that affects movement and muscle coordination. While the primary symptoms of CP are related to motor function, individuals with CP may also experience sensory impairments and perceptual difficulties. Let's discuss some of the common sensory impairments associated with CP, including visual and auditory impairments, as well as sensory processing difficulties.

1. Visual Impairment: Visual impairments are relatively common in individuals with CP. Conditions such as strabismus (crossed eyes), nystagmus (involuntary eye movements), or refractive errors may affect visual acuity. Some individuals may also have difficulty with visual perception, depth perception, or tracking objects with their eyes. Visual impairments can impact a person's ability to navigate the environment, recognize faces, or read.

2. Auditory Impairment: Hearing loss or auditory impairments can occur in individuals with CP. The causes of hearing impairment can be varied, including damage to the auditory nerves, ear infections, or structural abnormalities in the ear. These impairments can affect a person's ability to understand speech, localize sounds, and participate in auditory-based activities.

3. Sensory Processing Difficulties: Sensory processing difficulties are commonly observed in individuals with CP. Sensory processing refers to how the brain interprets and responds to sensory information from the environment. People with CP may experience sensory sensitivities or sensory-seeking behaviors. Sensory sensitivities may manifest as heightened sensitivity or aversion to certain stimuli, such as touch, sound, or light. On the other hand, sensory-seeking behaviors involve seeking out intense sensory input, such as spinning or rocking, to regulate sensory input.

   These sensory impairments and perceptual difficulties associated with CP can impact an individual's overall functioning and daily life. However, it is important to note that the specific nature and severity of these impairments can vary greatly among individuals with CP. Proper assessment and intervention by healthcare professionals, including occupational therapists, physical therapists, ophthalmologists, or audiologists, can help address and manage these sensory challenges. They may use strategies such as adaptive equipment, sensory integration therapy, or assistive technologies to enhance sensory experiences and promote overall well-being.

4.3 Intellectual and Learning Disabilities.

That's correct. While cerebral palsy (CP) primarily affects movement and muscle control, it's important to recognize that not all individuals with CP experience intellectual or learning disabilities. However, some individuals with CP may face cognitive challenges that can impact their learning and academic pursuits.

The cognitive challenges associated with CP can vary widely, as the condition affects each person differently. Here are a few examples of cognitive difficulties that individuals with CP may encounter:

1. Learning Disabilities: Some individuals with CP may have specific learning disabilities, such as difficulties with reading (dyslexia), writing (dysgraphia), or math (dyscalculia). These challenges can affect their ability to acquire and process information in traditional academic settings.
2. Executive Functioning: Executive functioning refers to a set of mental processes involved in planning, organizing, problem-solving, and self-regulation. Some individuals with CP may experience difficulties with executive functioning skills, making it harder for them to manage their time, set goals, stay organized, or initiate and complete tasks.
3. Processing Speed: Processing speed refers to the ability to efficiently and accurately process information. Some individuals with CP may have slower processing speed, which can affect their ability to quickly comprehend and respond to information presented in academic or everyday situations.
4. Memory and Attention: Difficulties with memory and attention can also impact learning in individuals with CP. They may have challenges with retaining and recalling information or struggle with sustained attention and focus, which can affect their ability to absorb new material and participate fully in academic activities.

   It is important to recognize that these cognitive challenges do not affect all individuals with CP, and the severity and specific areas of difficulty can vary from person to person. Additionally, many individuals with CP are highly capable and can thrive academically with appropriate accommodations, support, and individualized educational plans.

To address cognitive challenges in individuals with CP, a multidisciplinary approach involving educators, special education professionals, occupational therapists, and speech and language therapists can be beneficial. They can provide appropriate accommodations, assistive technologies, and tailored strategies to support learning and academic success based on the individual's unique needs and abilities.

Section 5: Emotional and Social Considerations:

5.1 Emotional Well-being

Living with cerebral palsy (CP) can have a significant emotional impact on individuals. The challenges and limitations associated with CP can give rise to frustration, self-esteem issues, and other emotional struggles. It is crucial to acknowledge and address these emotional aspects while providing appropriate mental health support.

1. Frustration: The physical limitations and barriers faced by individuals with CP can lead to frustration. Difficulties with mobility, communication, or activities of daily living can be frustrating, especially when they hinder independence or participation in desired activities. It's important to provide support and coping strategies to help individuals manage their frustration effectively.
2. Self-Esteem Issues: The visible differences or mobility challenges associated with CP can sometimes lead to self-esteem issues. Negative societal attitudes, stereotypes, or experiences of discrimination may also contribute to lower self-esteem. It's important to foster a positive self-image and promote self-acceptance by celebrating individual strengths, and accomplishments, and encouraging a supportive environment.
3. Mental Health Support: Individuals with CP may benefit from mental health support to address emotional challenges. Access to counseling, therapy, or support groups can provide a safe space to express feelings, develop coping strategies, and explore ways to enhance overall well-being. Mental health professionals can guide you in managing stress, building resilience, and addressing any specific emotional difficulties that arise.

   Supportive family and friends play a crucial role in the emotional well-being of individuals with CP. Encouragement, understanding, and open communication can make a positive difference. Additionally, raising awareness and promoting inclusion in society can help combat negative attitudes and provide opportunities for individuals with CP to lead fulfilling lives.

It's important to remember that mental health support is not only beneficial for individuals with CP but for their caregivers and family members as well. Coping with the challenges and responsibilities of caring for someone with CP can also be emotionally demanding, and seeking support is equally important for their well-being.

By addressing the emotional impact of living with CP and providing appropriate mental health support, we can contribute to the overall well-being and quality of life of individuals with CP and their support networks.

5.2 Social Interactions and Inclusion

Individuals with cerebral palsy (CP) may face challenges in social interaction due to their unique physical and communication abilities. These challenges can include difficulties with speech, mobility, and fine motor skills, which can affect their ability to engage in typical social interactions. It is crucial to create inclusive environments that foster acceptance and understanding to support their social participation and overall well-being.

1. Communication Barriers: Some individuals with CP may have speech difficulties or rely on alternative forms of communication such as augmentative and alternative communication (AAC) devices, sign language, or communication boards. Others may have difficulty with nonverbal communication, such as facial expressions or gestures. Others need to be patient, attentive, and open to alternative communication methods to ensure effective interaction.

2. Mobility Challenges: Individuals with CP may have limited mobility, use assistive devices such as wheelchairs or walkers, or have atypical movements. Physical barriers in the environment, such as inaccessible buildings or lack of accommodations, can hinder their participation in social activities. Creating inclusive environments with accessible infrastructure and removing physical barriers promotes equal opportunities for social engagement.

3. Attitudinal Barriers: Negative attitudes, stereotypes, and misconceptions about disability can create social barriers for individuals with CP. It is essential to promote acceptance, empathy, and understanding among peers, educators, and the wider community. Encouraging inclusive language, providing disability awareness training, and fostering an inclusive culture can help break down attitudinal barriers and create a supportive social environment.

4. Peer Acceptance and Social Integration: Peer acceptance and social integration are vital for individuals with CP to feel included and valued. Educators, parents, and community members can play a significant role in promoting inclusive social environments. Encouraging positive social interactions, facilitating peer support programs, and promoting inclusive activities can help foster friendships, social connections, and a sense of belonging.

   Creating inclusive environments that foster acceptance and understanding benefits not only individuals with CP but also the broader community. It promotes diversity, encourages empathy and compassion, and enriches everyone's experiences. By embracing the unique abilities and perspectives of individuals with CP, we can create a society that values inclusion and celebrates the contributions of all its members.

   Education, awareness campaigns, and advocating for inclusive policies can help create more inclusive communities. Additionally, organizations and support groups focused on disabilities can provide resources, information, and platforms for individuals with CP and their families to connect, share experiences, and find support.

   Ultimately, the goal is to create a society where individuals with CP can engage in social interactions without barriers, enjoy fulfilling relationships, and participate actively in all aspects of life.

2 UNLEASHING YOUR INNER STRENGTH: EMBRACING YOUR ABILITIES.

Introduction:

Living with cerebral palsy (CP) comes with unique challenges, but it also presents an opportunity to discover and unleash your inner strength. This chapter will explore strategies and perspectives that can empower individuals with CP to embrace their abilities, cultivate resilience, and live fulfilling life. By tapping into your inner strength, you can overcome obstacles, set and achieve goals, and lead a life filled with purpose and joy.

1. Embracing Self-Acceptance:

Embracing your abilities starts with accepting yourself as you are, CP and all. Acknowledge that your condition does not define your worth or potential. Embrace your unique strengths, talents, and qualities. Practice self-compassion, celebrate your accomplishments, and nurture a positive self-image.

2. Cultivating a Growth Mindset:

Adopting a growth mindset can transform how you approach challenges. Embrace the belief that your abilities and skills can be developed through effort and persistence. Develop a mindset that encourages continuous improvement, resilience, and a willingness to take on new experiences.

3. Setting Goals and Taking Action:

Define your aspirations and set meaningful goals. Identify areas of interest, whether they are academic, personal, or professional. Break your goals into manageable steps and create your plan of action. Use your support network to stay motivated and accountable. Remember that progress is a journey, and each step forward is an accomplishment.

4. Advocating for Yourself:

Become an advocate for your needs and rights. Learn about your rights under disability laws and regulations. Communicate your needs clearly and confidently, whether it's in education, employment, or accessing resources. Educate others about CP, dispel misconceptions, and promote inclusivity and accessibility. By advocating for yourself, you empower others to better understand and support you.

5. Building a Supportive Network:

   Surround yourself with a supportive network of family, friends, mentors, and professionals who believe in you and your abilities. Seek out disability-specific support groups or organizations to connect with individuals who share similar experiences. Share your challenges, seek advice, and offer support to others. Building a support network can provide encouragement, guidance, and a sense of belonging.

6. Developing Resilience:

   Resilience is a powerful tool in navigating the challenges of CP. Embrace setbacks as opportunities for growth, learn from failures, and adapt to changing circumstances. Practice self-care to maintain physical and emotional well-being. Engage in activities that bring you joy, reduce stress, and boost your resilience. Remember that resilience is a skill that can be nurtured and strengthened over time.

7. Celebrating Achievements:

   Take time to acknowledge and celebrate your achievements, no matter how small they may seem. Recognize the progress you've made, the barriers you've overcome, and the skills you've developed. Celebrate both personal milestones and professional accomplishments. Share your successes with others, inspire those around you, and take pride in your journey.

Conclusion:

Unleashing your inner strength and embracing your abilities with CP is a transformative process. By cultivating self-acceptance, adopting a growth mindset, setting goals, advocating for yourself, building a supportive network, developing resilience, and celebrating achievements, you can unlock your full potential. Remember that you possess unique talents and strengths that can positively impact your life and the lives of others. Embrace the journey of self-discovery and embrace the incredible person you are. Your inner strength is waiting to be unleashed.

3 NAVIGATING THE MEDICAL MAZE: TREATMENT OPTIONS AND THERAPIES.

Navigating the medical maze of treatment options and therapies for cerebral palsy (CP) can be complex. The management of CP typically involves a multidisciplinary approach that addresses the specific needs and goals of the individual. Here, we will discuss some common treatment options and therapies available for individuals with CP:

1. Physical Therapy (PT):

   Physical therapy plays a central role in managing CP. PT focuses on improving mobility, strength, coordination, and motor skills through exercises, stretches, and specialized techniques. Therapists work with individuals to address specific motor impairments and develop personalized treatment plans to enhance functional abilities.

2. Occupational Therapy (OT):

   Occupational therapy helps individuals with CP improve their independence in daily activities, such as self-care, fine motor skills, and sensory integration. OT aims to enhance functional abilities by using adaptive techniques, assistive devices, and modifications to the environment.

3. Speech and Language Therapy:

   Speech and language therapy focuses on improving communication skills, speech clarity, swallowing, and language development in individuals with CP who may experience speech and language difficulties. Therapists use various techniques, such as oral-motor exercises, augmentative and alternative communication (AAC) systems, and language interventions to enhance communication abilities.

4. Assistive Devices and Orthotics:

   Assistive devices and orthotics can play a crucial role in managing CP. These devices include wheelchairs, walkers, canes, and customized orthotic braces. They provide support, stability, and mobility assistance to help individuals with CP move more independently and participate in activities.

5. Medications:

   In some cases, medications may be prescribed to manage specific symptoms associated with CP. These medications can include muscle relaxants to reduce muscle stiffness and spasticity, anticonvulsants to manage seizures, or pain medications for discomfort or musculoskeletal issues. Medication use is typically determined on an individual basis and may require close monitoring by a healthcare professional.

6. Intrathecal Baclofen Therapy:

Intrathecal baclofen therapy involves the delivery of a muscle relaxant medication directly into the fluid surrounding the spinal cord through a surgically implanted pump. This therapy helps manage severe spasticity that is not effectively controlled by oral medications alone.

7. Botulinum Toxin Injections:

Botulinum toxin injections, commonly known as Botox injections, can be used to reduce muscle spasticity and improve range of motion. These injections are administered directly into specific muscles and can provide temporary relief from muscle stiffness and improve functional abilities.

8. Surgical Interventions:

In some cases, surgical interventions may be considered to improve mobility and correct structural abnormalities associated with CP. Surgeries can include muscle lengthening or tendon release procedures, joint stabilization, or orthopedic surgeries to correct skeletal deformities. These interventions are typically performed by specialized orthopedic surgeons.

9. Conductive Education:

Conductive Education is an educational and rehabilitative approach that focuses on improving movement, coordination, and independence. It combines physical and cognitive exercises in a structured group setting to promote motor learning and functional skills. Conductive Education programs are often conducted by specially trained conductors.

10. Hippotherapy:

Hippotherapy involves using horseback riding as a therapeutic tool for individuals with CP. The rhythmic movement of the horse can help improve balance, coordination, posture, and muscle strength. In addition to the physical benefits, the interaction with the horse can also have psychological and emotional benefits.

11. Aquatic Therapy:

Aquatic therapy, or hydrotherapy, utilizes the properties of water to support and assist with movement. The buoyancy of water reduces the effects of gravity and provides a low-impact environment for exercises and activities. Aquatic therapy can help improve muscle strength, flexibility, range of motion, and overall mobility.

12. Hyperbaric Oxygen Therapy (HBOT):

HBOT involves breathing pure oxygen in a pressurized chamber. It is believed to increase the amount of oxygen in the bloodstream, which can promote healing, reduce inflammation, and support tissue repair. Some individuals with CP may undergo HBOT as an adjunct therapy, although its effectiveness for CP is still a topic of debate and further research.

13. Constraint-Induced Movement Therapy (CIMT):

CIMT is a therapy approach that focuses on promoting the use of the affected limb by restricting the use of the unaffected limb. By restraining the unaffected limb and engaging in intensive therapy activities that encourage the use of the affected limb, individuals can improve motor function and regain more functional use of the affected limb.

14. Virtual Reality (VR) and Gaming:

Virtual reality and gaming technologies are increasingly being utilized in therapy for individuals with CP. These immersive experiences can engage and motivate individuals while targeting specific motor skills, balance, coordination, and cognitive abilities. VR and gaming can make therapy sessions more enjoyable and interactive, enhancing engagement and participation.

15. Alternative and Complementary Therapies:

Some individuals with CP may explore alternative or complementary therapies, such as acupuncture, massage therapy, chiropractic care, or nutritional interventions. These approaches can vary in effectiveness and should be discussed with healthcare professionals to ensure safety and to determine any potential benefits.

It is important to emphasize that not all therapies and treatment options are suitable or effective for every individual with CP. Each person's needs and responses to interventions may differ, and it is essential to consult with healthcare professionals to determine the most appropriate and evidence-based approaches.

Furthermore, ongoing research and advancements in medical technology continue to explore new treatment options and interventions for CP. Staying informed about emerging therapies and participating in clinical trials or research studies may provide individuals with CP access to innovative treatments.

Remember, the treatment journey for CP is highly individualized, and a collaborative approach involving healthcare professionals, therapists, caregivers, and the individual themselves is crucial in determining the most effective and comprehensive treatment plan.

4 ALLIES ON YOUR JOURNEY: BUILDING A SUPPORTIVE NETWORK.

Introduction:

Living with cerebral palsy (CP) can be both a rewarding and challenging journey. Building a supportive network of allies is essential in navigating the ups and downs that come with CP. This chapter explores the significance of allies and guides how to build a strong support system to empower and uplift individuals with CP.

1. Family and Caregivers:

   Family members and caregivers play a crucial role as allies in the journey of individuals with CP. They provide emotional support, advocacy, and practical assistance. Open and honest communication with family members is vital in fostering understanding and collaboration. Engaging family members in education and awareness about CP helps build a foundation of support.

2. Friends:

   Friends can be powerful allies in providing social support, companionship, and a sense of belonging. Encourage open conversations about CP with friends, allowing them to understand your experiences and challenges better. True friends will accept you for who you are, offer encouragement, and create inclusive environments where you can thrive.

3. Peers with CP:

   Connecting with peers who also have CP can be empowering. These individuals share similar experiences and understand the unique challenges faced. Joining support groups, attending CP-focused events, or participating in online communities can facilitate connections with peers, allowing for the exchange of advice, insights, and encouragement.

4. Medical Professionals:

   Developing a strong relationship with medical professionals who specialize in CP is crucial. These professionals, such as doctors, therapists, and specialists, provide expertise, guidance, and evidence-based interventions. Collaborate with them to create personalized treatment plans, seek second opinions when needed, and stay informed about advancements in CP management.

5. Educators and School Staff:

   In the educational setting, educators and school staff can be valuable allies. Communicate openly about your needs, accommodations, and goals. Work with teachers to ensure a supportive learning environment that fosters inclusivity and enables academic success. Educate them about CP and provide resources to enhance their understanding.

6. Advocacy Groups and Organizations:

   Connect with advocacy groups and organizations that focus on CP. These groups provide a wealth of resources, support, and opportunities for networking. They advocate for the rights of individuals with CP, raise awareness, and offer platforms for education, empowerment, and collaboration.

7. Mentors and Role Models:

   Seek out mentors and role models who have successfully navigated their journey with CP or other disabilities. They can provide guidance, inspiration, and practical advice. Engage in mentoring programs, join mentorship networks, or reach out to individuals you admire for mentorship opportunities.

8. Online Communities:

   The internet offers a vast array of online communities, forums, and social media platforms where individuals with CP can connect and share experiences. Engaging with these communities can provide a sense of belonging, valuable insights, and emotional support from individuals who truly understand the challenges and triumphs of living with CP.

9. Supportive Professionals:

   Beyond medical professionals, various supportive professionals can aid in your journey with CP. These may include social workers, psychologists, counselors, or life coaches. Seek their expertise to address emotional well-being, coping strategies, goal-setting, and enhancing the overall quality of life.

Conclusion:

Building a supportive network of allies is a transformative step in the journey of individuals with CP. Allies provide encouragement, understanding, and practical support. By nurturing relationships with family, friends, peers, medical professionals, educators, advocates, mentors, and online communities, you create a strong foundation of support, empowerment, and inclusivity. Remember, you are not alone on this journey, and together with your allies, you can overcome challenges, celebrate achievements, and embrace a fulfilling life with CP.

5 OVERCOMING OBSTACLES: STRATEGIES FOR EVERYDAY CHALLENGES.

INTRODUCTION

Living with cerebral palsy presents individuals with a unique set of challenges in their daily lives. However, with the right strategies and support, these obstacles can be overcome. This chapter aims to provide practical strategies for people with cerebral palsy to navigate everyday challenges. By implementing these strategies, individuals can enhance their independence, improve their quality of life, and overcome barriers effectively.

1. Mobility and Accessibility Challenges:

   One of the significant obstacles faced by individuals with cerebral palsy is mobility and accessibility. Here are some strategies to overcome these challenges:

   a. Assistive Devices: Utilize assistive devices such as wheelchairs, walkers, canes, or orthotics to enhance mobility and independence. Consult with a healthcare professional to determine the most suitable device for your specific needs.

   b. Home Modifications: Make necessary modifications to your living environment to improve accessibility. Install ramps, grab bars, and widen doorways to accommodate wheelchairs and walkers. Rearrange furniture to create wider pathways for easier navigation.

   c. Accessible Transportation: Seek accessible transportation options such as wheelchair-accessible vans, public transit services with ramps or lifts, or specialized transportation services for people with disabilities.

2. Communication and Social Interaction Challenges:

   Cerebral palsy can sometimes present challenges in communication and social interactions. Here are strategies to help overcome these obstacles:

   a. Augmentative and Alternative Communication (AAC) Systems: Utilize AAC systems such as communication boards, speech-generating devices, or mobile applications to support communication. Work with a speech-language pathologist to identify the most effective AAC system for your needs.

   b. Speech Therapy: Engage in regular speech therapy sessions to improve speech articulation and clarity. Speech therapists can provide exercises and techniques tailored to your specific challenges.

c. Social Skills Training: Participate in social skills training programs to enhance social interaction abilities. These programs can offer guidance on initiating conversations, understanding social cues, and building relationships.

3. Independence and Daily Living Challenges:

Independence in daily activities is crucial for individuals with cerebral palsy. The following strategies can help overcome challenges and promote independence:

a. Adaptive Equipment and Assistive Technology: Utilize adaptive equipment and assistive technology designed for specific tasks. Examples include modified utensils, dressing aids, and voice-activated smart home devices. These tools can facilitate independent living and reduce dependence on others.

b. Occupational Therapy: Engage in occupational therapy sessions to develop skills for daily living activities. Occupational therapists can guide you in improving fine motor skills, developing self-care routines, and adapting activities to your abilities.

c. Time Management and Organization: Implement strategies for effective time management and organization. Use tools like calendars, planners, and reminders on your phone or computer to keep track of tasks and appointments.

4. Emotional and Psychological Challenges:

Living with cerebral palsy can sometimes lead to emotional and psychological challenges. Here are strategies to address these issues:

a. Support Network: Build a strong support network consisting of family, friends, and support groups. Surround yourself with individuals who understand and empathize with your experiences.

b. Counseling and Therapy: Seek counseling or therapy from mental health professionals who specialize in working with individuals with disabilities. They can provide stress management, and build resilience.

c. Self-Care and Stress Reduction: Prioritize self-care activities to promote emotional well-being. Engage in relaxation techniques, such as deep breathing exercises, meditation, or engaging in hobbies that bring joy and relaxation.

Conclusion:

Overcoming obstacles faced by individuals with cerebral palsy requires a proactive approach, utilizing appropriate strategies and support systems. By implementing the strategies discussed in this chapter, individuals can enhance their independence, communication skills, and overall quality of life. Remember that each person's journey is unique, and it's essential to tailor these strategies to your specific needs and goals. With determination, resilience, and the right support, you can overcome the challenges posed by cerebral palsy and lead a fulfilling life.

Remember, it's crucial to work closely with a team of healthcare professionals, including doctors, therapists, and specialists who can provide personalized guidance and support. They can help you identify additional strategies, monitor your progress, and make necessary adjustments along the way.

Furthermore, don't hesitate to advocate for yourself and your needs. You have the right to access equal opportunities and accommodations. Be vocal about your requirements in various settings, such as educational institutions, workplaces, and public spaces. By asserting your needs and educating others about cerebral palsy, you can contribute to a more inclusive and understanding society.

Lastly, never underestimate the power of a positive mindset. While challenges may arise, maintaining a positive outlook can significantly impact your ability to overcome obstacles. Surround yourself with positive influences, celebrate your achievements, and remind yourself of your strengths and capabilities.

Living with cerebral palsy may present challenges, but with the right strategies, support, and mindset, you can overcome them. Embrace your journey, celebrate your progress, and keep pushing forward. Remember, you are not defined by your disability, but by the strength, determination, and resilience you demonstrate every day.

By implementing these strategies and adopting a proactive approach, individuals with cerebral palsy can overcome obstacles, and seize opportunities.

6 ADAPTIVE TECHNOLOGY: TOOLS TO EMPOWER YOUR INDEPENDENCE.

Introduction:

Living with cerebral palsy presents unique challenges, but thanks to advancements in technology, individuals with this condition have access to a wide range of adaptive tools and devices that can significantly enhance their independence and quality of life. In this chapter, we will explore various adaptive technologies specifically designed to address the needs of individuals with cerebral palsy. These tools aim to assist with mobility, communication, daily tasks, education, and recreation, ultimately empowering individuals with cerebral palsy to lead more independent lives.

Section 1: Mobility Aids

1.1 Wheelchairs and Mobility Scooters:

- Power wheelchairs: These electric-powered wheelchairs provide enhanced mobility and maneuverability for individuals with limited upper body strength or control.
- Manual wheelchairs: Lightweight and customizable, manual wheelchairs offer individuals the flexibility to propel themselves independently or with minimal assistance.
- Mobility scooters: These devices are ideal for individuals with cerebral palsy who have limited mobility but can still stand and walk short distances. Scooters provide a convenient and efficient means of transportation.

1.2 Walkers and Gait Trainers:

- Standard walkers: Designed for individuals who require minimal support, walkers offer stability and balance assistance during walking.
- Gait trainers: These devices provide a more comprehensive solution by offering support for those with more severe mobility impairments. Gait trainers are adjustable and often come with features such as supportive harnesses and swivel wheels.

1.3 Walkers and Gait Trainers:

- Ankle-foot orthoses (AFOs): AFOs provide support and stabilization to the lower limbs, helping individuals with spasticity or difficulties in foot positioning to maintain proper alignment while walking or standing.

- Canes and crutches: These devices offer additional support during walking, helping individuals with cerebral palsy maintain balance and stability.

Section 2: Communication Aids

2.1 Augmentative and Alternative Communication (AAC) Devices:

- Speech-generating devices: These devices enable individuals with speech difficulties to express themselves using pre-programmed phrases, symbols, or synthesized voices.
- Communication boards: A low-tech alternative, communication boards consist of pictures, symbols, or text that individuals can point to communicate their needs or desires.

2.2 Eye-Gaze Systems:

- Eye-tracking devices: These systems use specialized cameras to track eye movements and convert them into commands, allowing individuals with limited mobility or speech to control computers, communication devices, or environmental controls.

Section 3: Daily Living Aids

3.1 Adaptive Utensils and Tools:

- Modified utensils: Designed with larger handles, built-up grips, or angled designs, these utensils enable individuals with limited dexterity or hand control to feed themselves more easily.
- Adaptive tools: Devices such as button hooks, zipper pulls, and reaching aids assist individuals with cerebral palsy in managing daily tasks independently.

3.2 Environmental Control Systems:

- Home automation: With voice-activated or remote-controlled systems, individuals with limited mobility can control lights, thermostats, appliances, and security systems.
- Smart home devices: Smart speakers and home assistants like Amazon Alexa or Google Home can help individuals with cerebral palsy access information, make phone calls, set reminders, and perform various tasks using voice commands.

Section 4: Education and Recreation Aids

4.1 Assistive Technology in Education:

- Computer software: Specialized educational software can assist individuals with cerebral palsy in reading, writing, and organizing information.
- Alternative input devices: Switches, touchscreens, or eye-tracking systems can enable individuals with physical impairments to access computers and educational materials.

4.2 Adaptive Gaming Devices:

- Accessible gaming controllers: These controllers are designed with larger buttons, customizable layouts, and alternative input methods to accommodate individuals with limited dexterity or mobility.
- Switch interfaces: Switch interfaces allow individuals to play games using external switches, which can be operated by various body parts, such as hands, feet, or head movements.

4.3 Recreational Adaptations:

- Adaptive sports equipment: From modified bicycles and tricycles to specialized sports wheelchairs, adaptive sports equipment enables individuals with cerebral palsy to participate in various recreational activities.
- Adaptive art and music tools: Adapted art tools, such as specially designed brushes or grips, and musical instruments with modified keys or switches, allow individuals with cerebral palsy to engage in creative expression.

Conclusion:

Adaptive technology has revolutionized the lives of individuals with cerebral palsy, providing them with tools and devices that promote independence, enhance mobility, facilitate communication, and enable participation in various daily activities, education, and recreation. By harnessing the power of technology, individuals with cerebral palsy can overcome physical limitations and unlock their full potential, leading fulfilling and independent lives. As technology continues to advance, it holds the promise of further empowering individuals with cerebral palsy, opening up new possibilities and opportunities for a brighter future.

7 ADVOCATING FOR YOURSELF: MAKING YOUR VOICE HEARD.

Advocating for yourself and making your voice heard is essential for anyone, including individuals with cerebral palsy. Cerebral palsy is a condition that affects a person's movement, muscle control, and coordination. However, it does not diminish a person's ability to express their thoughts, desires, and needs. Here are some strategies and tips to help you advocate for yourself effectively:

1. Educate Yourself: Gain a thorough understanding of your rights, the challenges you may face, and the available resources. Learn about laws and regulations that protect the rights of individuals with disabilities, such as the Americans with Disabilities Act (ADA) in the United States or similar legislation in your country.
2. Know Your Strengths and Limitations: Be aware of your strengths and limitations, as well as your specific needs related to cerebral palsy. Understanding your abilities will enable you to communicate your needs more effectively and request reasonable accommodations when necessary.
3. Develop Self-Confidence: Build your self-confidence by focusing on your accomplishments and strengths. Recognize that your voice and experiences are valuable. Surround yourself with supportive individuals who uplift and encourage you.
4. Communicate Your Needs: Clearly and assertively communicate your needs and preferences to others. Be specific about what you require to maximize your potential and participate fully in activities or situations. Use straightforward language and be prepared to explain if necessary.
5. Seek Supportive Allies: Build a network of supportive individuals who can help amplify your voice. This may include family members, friends, healthcare professionals, educators, or disability advocacy groups. They can provide guidance, advice, and assistance in navigating challenges.
6. Utilize Assistive Technology: Depending on your individual needs, consider utilizing assistive technology to enhance your communication abilities. This may include speech-generating devices, communication apps, alternative and augmentative communication (AAC) methods, or other tools that aid in expressing your thoughts and ideas.

7. Stay Informed: Keep up-to-date with advancements, research, and new technologies related to cerebral palsy. Being informed empowers you to make informed decisions, understand potential treatments or interventions, and advocate for yourself from an informed standpoint.
8. Practice Self-Advocacy: Actively engage in self-advocacy by speaking up for yourself in various settings, such as educational institutions, workplaces, healthcare settings, or social environments. Remember, you have the right to be heard and respected.
9. Document Your Experiences: Maintain a record of any discriminatory incidents, challenges faced, or instances where accommodations were denied. This documentation can serve as evidence if you need to escalate a situation or file a complaint.
10. Connect with Supportive Organizations: Seek out organizations or groups that specifically focus on cerebral palsy or disability advocacy. These groups can provide valuable resources, support, and opportunities for networking with individuals who share similar experiences.

Remember, advocating for yourself is an ongoing process, and it may take time to develop effective strategies. Don't hesitate to seek assistance when needed, and remember that your voice matters. By speaking up, you can help create positive change and ensure that your needs are met.

8 INSPIRING OTHERS: SHARING YOUR STORY AND MAKING A POSITIVE IMPACT.

Introduction:

Having cerebral palsy gives you a unique perspective on life and the challenges you face. By sharing your story and experiences, you have the power to inspire others and make a positive impact in their lives. This chapter explores the importance of sharing your story, offers tips on how to effectively communicate your experiences, and provides guidance on how to create a positive impact in the lives of others.

1. Embrace Your Story:

a. Reflect on your journey with cerebral palsy and recognize the strength, resilience, and lessons you have gained from your experiences.

b. Embrace your story, including both the triumphs and the challenges. Understand that sharing your vulnerabilities can be empowering and relatable.

2. Find Your Motivation:

Identify your motivation for sharing your story. Are you hoping to raise awareness, provide support, or inspire others? Understanding your purpose will guide your storytelling approach.

3. Craft Your Narrative:

a. Determine the key messages you want to convey through your story. Consider the aspects of your experience that you believe will resonate with others and have the most significant impact.

b. Structure your narrative by incorporating a compelling introduction, a well-developed middle section that delves into the details of your journey, and a powerful conclusion that leaves a lasting impression.

4. Choose Your Platforms:

a. Identify the platforms and mediums through which you want to share your story. This could include public speaking engagements, social media, blogs, vlogs, or writing articles for publications.

b. Consider your target audience and select platforms that will effectively reach and engage with them.

5. Utilize Social Media:
    a. Leverage social media platforms to share your story, raise awareness, and connect with others. Utilize hashtags related to cerebral palsy and disability advocacy to expand your reach.
    b. Engage with your audience by responding to comments, messages, and questions, fostering a supportive community.
6. Be Authentic and Vulnerable:
    a. Share your story authentically, allowing yourself to be vulnerable. This creates a genuine connection with your audience and makes your experiences relatable.
    b. Don't be afraid to discuss the challenges you've faced, as well as the strategies and mindset that helped you overcome them.
7. Educate and Inform:
    a. Use your storytelling as an opportunity to educate others about cerebral palsy and debunk misconceptions. Provide accurate information about the condition, its impact, and available support resources.
    b. Share your insights and strategies for managing daily life, such as adaptive equipment, therapies, or community support networks
8. Inspire and Empower:
    a. Share the successes and achievements you've experienced despite the challenges of cerebral palsy. Highlight the milestones, personal growth, and moments of triumph that inspire hope and resilience.
    b. Encourage and empower others by emphasizing the importance of self-acceptance, self-advocacy, and pursuing their dreams despite obstacles.
9. Collaborate and Connect:
    a. Collaborate with other individuals and organizations in the disability community to amplify your impact. Seek opportunities to partner on advocacy projects, events, or initiatives that align with your values and goals.
    b. Connect with individuals who resonate with your story and engage in meaningful conversations to foster a sense of community and support.

10. Measure Your Impact:

a. Reflect on the impact you're making through feedback, comments, and personal stories shared by those who have been influenced by your experiences.
b. Keep track of the opportunities that arise from sharing your story, such as speaking engagements, partnerships, or invitations to contribute to publications.

Conclusion:

By sharing your story and experiences, you have the power to inspire, educate, and create a positive impact in the lives of others.

9 EXPLORING DREAMS AND GOALS: SETTING AND ACHIEVING PERSONAL MILESTONES.

Introduction:

Living with cerebral palsy (CP) does not diminish your ability to dream big, set goals, and achieve personal milestones. It can provide you with the determination and resilience needed to overcome challenges and pursue your passions. This chapter focuses on exploring dreams and goals, setting realistic milestones, and providing strategies to help you achieve them.

1. Reflect on Your Passions:
    a. Take the time to reflect on your interests, talents, and passions. Consider what activities or pursuits bring you joy, fulfillment, and a sense of purpose.
    b. Identify areas where you feel motivated to make progress, whether it's in education, career, relationships, creative endeavors, or personal growth.
2. Set Realistic and Measurable Goals:
    a. Break down your long-term dreams into smaller, achievable goals. This will help you stay motivated and focused along the way.
    b. Ensure that your goals are specific, measurable, attainable, relevant, and time-bound (SMART). This framework will help you create a clear roadmap for success.
3. Seek Support and Guidance:
    a. Reach out to supportive individuals in your life, such as family, friends, mentors, or professionals, who can provide guidance and encouragement.
    b. Connect with disability-specific organizations or support groups that can offer resources, networking opportunities, and advice from individuals who have similar experiences.
4. Develop an Action Plan:
    a. Create a detailed action plan outlining the steps you need to take to achieve each goal. Break down each goal into smaller, manageable tasks and assign deadlines to hold yourself accountable.
    b. Consider any accommodations or adaptations you may require to overcome physical or logistical challenges. Research assistive technologies, adaptive equipment, or support services that can help you in pursuing your goals.

5. Build a Strong Support System:
    a. Surround yourself with people who believe in your abilities and aspirations. Cultivate a support system that encourages and motivates you to overcome obstacles.
    b. Seek out mentors or role models who have achieved similar goals or who can provide valuable insights and advice.
6. Embrace a Growth Mindset:
    a. Adopt a growth mindset that recognizes challenges as opportunities for learning and growth. Embrace the belief that with effort, perseverance, and adaptability, you can overcome obstacles and make progress.
    b. View setbacks or failures as valuable lessons and stepping stones toward success, rather than as reasons to give up.
7. Celebrate Milestones:
    a. Acknowledge and celebrate your achievements along the way, no matter how small. Recognize the progress you've made and the efforts you've invested.
    b. Use milestones as opportunities to reflect on your journey, re-evaluate your goals if necessary, and set new challenges to continue your personal growth.
8. Practice Self-Care:
    a. Take care of your physical and emotional well-being. Engage in activities that promote self-care, such as exercise, mindfulness, hobbies, and spending time with loved ones.
    b. Prioritize rest and recovery to ensure you have the energy and focus to pursue your goals with vigor.
9. Seek Opportunities for Growth:
    a. Continuously seek opportunities for learning and growth. Attend workshops, conferences, or educational programs related to your areas of interest.
    b. Step out of your comfort zone and explore new experiences that challenge you and expand your horizons.
10. Inspire Others:
    a. Share your journey and achievements with others to inspire and empower them. Your story can be a source of motivation for others facing similar challenges.
    b. Use your experiences to advocate for inclusivity, accessibility, and equal opportunities

for individuals with disabilities.

Conclusion:

Living with cerebral palsy should not hinder you from pursuing your dreams and setting personal milestones. By reflecting on your passions, setting realistic goals, seeking support, and adopting a growth mindset, you can overcome challenges and achieve personal milestones. Remember to celebrate your achievements and practice self-care along the way. By sharing your journey and inspiring others, you can make a lasting impact and contribute to a more inclusive society. Your dreams are within reach, and with determination and perseverance, you can turn them into reality.

10 A BRIGHT FUTURE: TRANSITIONING INTO ADULTHOOD WITH CEREBRAL PALSY.

Introduction:

Transitioning into adulthood is an exciting and transformative phase of life, filled with new opportunities, challenges, and possibilities. For individuals with cerebral palsy (CP), this transition may involve unique considerations and preparations. This chapter explores the key aspects of transitioning into adulthood with CP, providing guidance and strategies to embrace a bright future.

1. Self-Exploration and Identity:
    a. Engage in self-reflection to gain a deeper understanding of your identity, values, interests, and aspirations. This self-awareness will guide your decisions and choices as you transition into adulthood.
    b. Embrace your identity as a person with CP, recognizing it as a part of who you are while understanding that it does not define your entire being.
2. Education and Career Planning:
    a. Assess your educational goals and aspirations. Explore various educational pathways and resources available to you, such as inclusive schools, vocational programs, or higher education institutions.
    b. Seek guidance from career counselors, mentors, or disability support services to explore career options that align with your interests, strengths, and abilities. Consider potential accommodations or adaptations that may be necessary in the workplace.
3. Independent Living Skills:
    a. Develop practical skills for independent living, such as managing finances, cooking, cleaning, transportation, and personal care. Seek training, if needed, to enhance your abilities in these areas.
    b. Explore assistive technologies and adaptive equipment that can facilitate greater independence in daily activities.
4. Healthcare and Self-Advocacy:
    a. Transitioning into adulthood involves taking charge of your healthcare. Familiarize

yourself with your medical history, medications, and any specific healthcare needs related to your CP.

b. Advocate for your healthcare needs by actively participating in medical decisions, seeking second opinions when necessary, and staying informed about new treatment options or therapies.

5. Building Support Networks:

a. Cultivate a support network of family, friends, mentors, and professionals who understand and support your goals and aspirations. They can provide guidance, encouragement, and connections to opportunities.

b. Connect with disability-specific organizations or support groups that can offer resources, mentorship, and networking opportunities with individuals who share similar experiences.

6. Financial Planning:

a. Begin planning for your financial future by exploring options such as disability benefits, scholarships, grants, or vocational rehabilitation programs that may provide financial support for education, employment, or independent living.

b. Seek advice from financial advisors or experts who can help you navigate financial planning, savings, budgeting, and accessing available resources.

7. Social Inclusion and Relationships:

a. Foster social connections and friendships with a diverse group of individuals. Participate in community activities, sports, clubs, or organizations that align with your interests and allow for social interaction.

b. Develop healthy and meaningful relationships, both romantic and platonic, by communicating your needs, expectations, and boundaries openly and honestly.

8. Self-Care and Well-Being:

a. Prioritize self-care and well-being as you navigate the transition into adulthood. Engage in activities that promote physical, mental, and emotional well-being, such as exercise, hobbies, mindfulness, and therapy.

b. Seek support from professionals or therapists who can assist with managing stress, anxiety, or any emotional challenges that may arise during this period.

9. Embracing Opportunities and Challenges:

a. Approach opportunities and challenges with a positive mindset and a willingness to learn and grow. Embrace new experiences, take calculated risks, and step out of your comfort zone to expand your horizons.

b. Use setbacks or obstacles as opportunities for personal growth and resilience. Seek support and guidance when needed, and remember that every experience contributes to your journey.

10. Advocating for Inclusivity and Accessibility:

a. As you transition into adulthood, advocate for inclusivity and accessibility in all aspects of life. Share your experiences and insights to raise awareness about the barriers individuals with CP may face and promote positive change.

b. Engage with advocacy organizations, participate in disability rights movements, and collaborate with like-minded individuals to create a more inclusive society for people with disabilities.

Conclusion:

Transitioning into adulthood with cerebral palsy is a transformative journey filled with opportunities for growth, self-discovery, and achievement. By exploring your identity, setting educational and career goals, developing independent living skills, building support networks, and prioritizing self-care, you can embrace a bright future. Remember to advocate for inclusivity and accessibility, and be open to the opportunities and challenges that come your way. With determination, resilience, and a positive mindset, you can create a fulfilling and meaningful life as you navigate the path to adulthood with cerebral palsy.

11 SOME KEY HISTORICAL BACKGROUND AND MILESTONES RELATED TO CEREBRAL PALSY

1. Ancient references:

While the term "cerebral palsy" did not exist in ancient times, there are historical references suggesting the presence of the condition. For example, ancient Egyptian hieroglyphs depict individuals with physical disabilities, potentially including cerebral palsy.

2. Early medical descriptions:

The earliest medical descriptions of cerebral palsy date back to the 19th century. In 1861, an English surgeon named William Little published a series of papers describing a group of children with movement difficulties and attributing the condition to birth-related brain damage.

3. The term "cerebral palsy":

The term "cerebral palsy" was first used in 1889 by Sir William Osler, a Canadian physician. He coined the term to describe the motor impairments resulting from brain damage in early childhood.

4. Advancements in understanding:

Throughout the 20th century, there were significant advancements in understanding cerebral palsy. Researchers, such as Sigmund Freud, Jean-Martin Charcot, and William G. Lennox, made contributions to the understanding of the condition's causes and characteristics.

5. Medical and therapeutic interventions:

In the mid-20th century, advancements in medical and therapeutic interventions began to emerge. These included the development of orthopedic surgeries, such as tendon lengthening or transfers, aimed at improving mobility and reducing muscle spasticity. Additionally, physiotherapy, occupational therapy, and speech therapy became integral parts of cerebral palsy treatment.

6. Deinstitutionalization movement:

In the 1960s and 1970s, a movement known as deinstitutionalization gained momentum. This movement aimed to shift care for individuals with cerebral palsy and other disabilities from large institutions to community-based settings, promoting a more inclusive and integrated approach.

7. Assistive technology:

The late 20th century witnessed significant advancements in assistive technology for individuals with cerebral palsy. Augmentative and alternative communication (AAC) devices, orthotic devices, powered wheelchairs, and computer-based assistive technologies have greatly enhanced the independence and quality of life of people with cerebral palsy.

8. Inclusive education:

Over the past few decades, there has been a growing emphasis on inclusive education for children with cerebral palsy. Efforts have been made to provide equal educational opportunities and promote integration into mainstream classrooms, with appropriate support and accommodations.

9. Neuroplasticity research:

In recent years, there has been an increased focus on neuroplasticity—the brain's ability to reorganize and adapt—to develop new approaches for cerebral palsy management. Research in this area explores interventions such as constraint-induced movement therapy, brain stimulation techniques, and emerging technologies like brain-computer interfaces.

10. Advocacy and awareness:

Cerebral palsy advocacy organizations and initiatives have played a crucial role in raising awareness, promoting research, and advocating for the rights and inclusion of individuals with cerebral palsy. Their efforts have contributed to shifting societal attitudes, improving accessibility, and fostering a more inclusive society.

These milestones highlight the evolving understanding, medical interventions, societal changes, and advancements in the management of cerebral palsy over time.

ABOUT THE AUTHOR

Vanessa A. Ray is a passionate advocate for individuals with disabilities, with a particular focus on cerebral palsy. Motivated by a deep understanding of the challenges and triumphs faced by those living with cerebral palsy, Vanessa has worked closely with medical professionals, therapists, and organizations to promote inclusivity, accessibility, and equal opportunities for individuals with disabilities.

Through her writing, Vanessa aims to share knowledge, insights, and practical guidance to navigate the journey of cerebral palsy. She is committed to raising awareness, promoting understanding, and inspiring hope among readers of "Little Warriors Guide to Cerebral Palsy."

Vanessa is grateful for the opportunity to contribute to the lives of little warriors and their families through this book. she hopes that her words will empower and inspire readers, fostering a greater understanding and appreciation for the unique journeys and abilities of individuals with cerebral palsy.

Printed in Great Britain
by Amazon

52557997R00031